Clean Eating Blueprint

A New Start for Your Healthy Body

By Cathy Wilson
Copyright © 2013

Income Disclaimer

This book contains business strategies, marketing methods and other business advice that, regardless of my own results and experience, may not produce the same results (or any results) for you. I make absolutely no guarantee, expressed or implied, that by following the advice below you will make any money or improve current profits, as there are several factors and variables that come into play regarding any given business.

Primarily, results will depend on the nature of the product or business model, the conditions of the marketplace, the experience of the individual, and situations and elements that are beyond your control.

As with any business endeavor, you assume all risk related to investment and money based on your own discretion and at your own potential expense.

Liability Disclaimer

By reading this book, you assume all risks associated with using the advice given below, with a full understanding that you, solely, are responsible for anything that may occur as a result of putting this information into action in any way, and regardless of your interpretation of the advice.

You further agree that our company cannot be held responsible in any way for the success or failure of your business as a result of the information presented in this book. It is your responsibility to conduct your own due diligence regarding the safe and successful operation of your business if you intend to apply any of our information in any way to your business operations.

Terms of Use

You are given a non-transferable, "personal use" license to this book. You cannot distribute it or share it with other individuals.

Also, there are no resale rights or private label rights granted when purchasing this book. In other words, it's for your own personal use only.

Clean Eating Blueprint

A New Start for Your Healthy Body

By Cathy Wilson

Table of Contents

Introduction

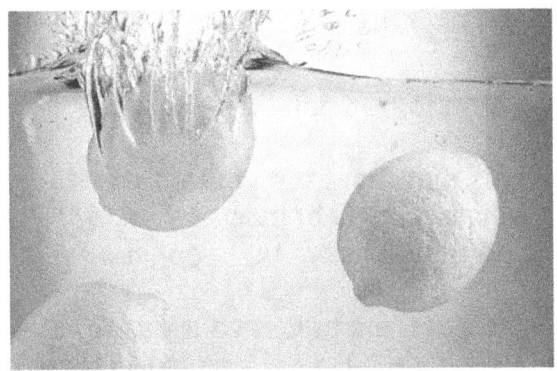

Is your health important to you?

Will you commit to detoxifying, restoring and re-energizing your body and mind to be rewarded with less disease, decreased chronic disease symptoms, less fat, increased energy, sharper cognitive skills and a more positive life attitude?

Clean Eating Blueprint is all about restoring control in your good health. It's important to understand first what's causing your energy to be depleted and serious disease to strike. Learning about how harmful our environment really is and how to change this is going to set you on the path to living a clean and healthy life with energy coming out of your ears! It's a breath of FRESH air, you might say.

The idea is to establish the blueprint to good clean eating and marrying it to your tolerances, preferences and life-style in general. The truth is there is no one black and white eating plan that is PERFECT for everyone. What you need to do is look for an eating strategy or concept that works for you and fit it into your life, striving for mental, physical, emotional and social balance.

Is it ever going to be perfect? Nope.

Is it always going to be changing? Yes it is.

Just as today is different from yesterday, your good health and wellness, weight loss and ability to stay disease-free is going to always be in constant motion.

This means you get you adjust your eating, exercise and other healthy lifestyle habits as you see fit, not necessarily what a specific eating plan dictates. Does this make sense? The Clean Eating Blueprint gives you detoxified bodily systems from which to build clean eating, fitness and lifestyle actions that will manifest into habits to give you a long and healthy life.

As a health and nutrition expert for over 20 years, I've learned through trial and error and working with other health professionals, that digging to the root of the problem is the only way to get things fixed. Otherwise you're just putting a band aid on the issue more often than not and all this is does is cause further interference in your well-being.

Let's have a look at the basic of clean eating and all that it reflects, with the goal of gaining the knowledge and "know-how" to help you lose weight, gain energy, avoid disease and "Get Clean!"

Who doesn't want to have their oil changed and premium fuel put in?

What is Clean Eating?

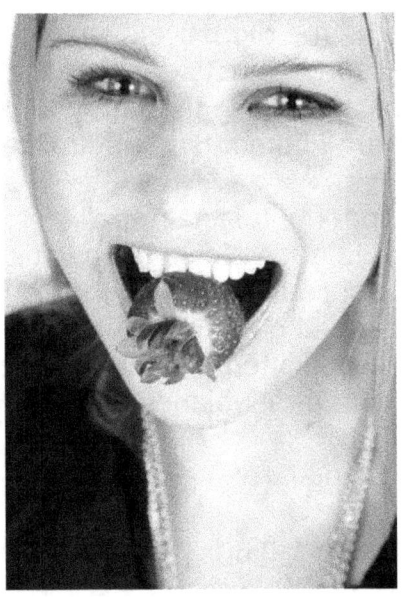

Clean eating is the concept and application of getting back to the basics, natural, healthy, clean eating that encourages your mental and physical to exist in perfect harmony. That may be a little "flowery", but you get the idea.

Clean eating is giving you the ability to purge your internal systems of poisonous toxins that are interfering with your good health and well-being. There are toxins that accumulate over time to trigger illness and disease that will steal your quality of life and eventually your life. Cancers, mental illness, cardiovascular disease, diabetes and stroke are just a few that are interconnected with the unhealthy environment with which we are associated.

You can ignore this or stand up and take action because you care about your health and about YOU.

Clean eating will help your body to:

.
* Relieve stress on the digestive system
* Improve protection against serious disease triggered by poisonous toxins circulating through your body
* Introduce powerful nutrients to neutralize debilitating liver toxins
* Trigger and support intestinal repair
This introduction to eating includes a liquid meal morning and night, with a solid meal during the day. The program has meals spaced out strategically so your overworked digestive system is allotted the time it needs to detoxify and restore to its natural balance.

The three focal points are:
* Detoxifying
* Restoring or Replenishing
* Re-energizing

By Detoxifying you'll eat organic and all-natural foods, get rid of bad bacteria in your system and look to steer clear of any harmful processed and packaged foods.

By Replenishing you'll load your system with essential vitamins and minerals, replenishing what has been de-pleted and making sure there are ample nutrients readily available to run your system optimally. Supplements will help to restore if you don't get the nutrients through food and getting at least 10-15 minutes of unprotected sun-light. EVERY day is going to give you the vitamin D you need to deter cancer and strengthen bones. Take note that eating clean and naturally should give your body all the nutrition it requires.

By Re-energizing all facets of life and taking care of you, optimal health and clean living will be restored. This includes regular maintenance through massages, saunas, relaxing mediation, and making sure you get enough fiber to keep yourself regular. It's a much needed method of maintenance and detoxifying the way nature intended.

There are recommended foods to eat throughout this Clean Eating Diet, along with daily exercise including as much walking and stair climbing as you can. It's best to get at least 30-45 minutes in per day, but anything is better than nothing. What's important is you understand the more exercise you get, both cardiovascular, strength and weight training, the more calories you will use, the more weight you will lose and the stronger, leaner and more energized you will feel.

Clean Eating makes sense and ideally it's something you should continue on with indefinitely, although modified to fit YOU a little more. Your absolute goal should be to always try and make better eating, exercise and living decisions always.

Does this mean you are always going to be perfect? Nope.

Is it okay to veer off course everyone once in a while? Absolutely!

It's all about give and take, learning and growing and enjoying every single day you are on this planet. You are the one that has to answer to you. This means that only you know what's best for you, or at least you get to figure that out.

My Thinking . . .

Clean eating is a choice. You can either decide to do it or not. The benefits are straight forward and clear. The tools to make this change for life will be uncovered. I can lead you to the water, but I can't make you drink even if you are dehydrated and dying of thirst.
The choice is yours.

Is the Environment Poisoning Us?

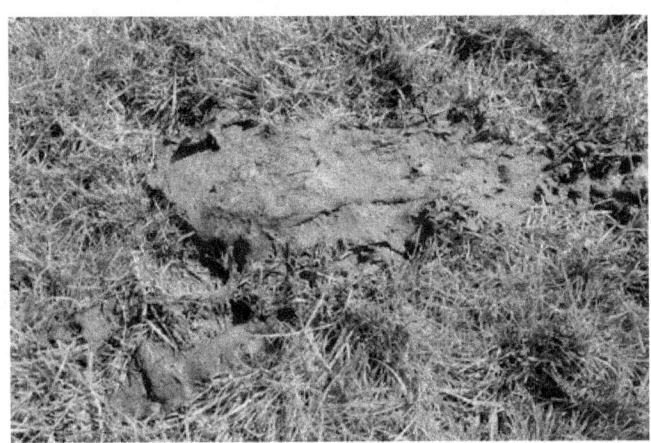

In short the answer is yes. We not only breathe and absorb harmful environmental toxins through our skin, but
we also ingest them through food. Waste from manufac-
turing and agricultural practices seep into streams, lakes,
rivers, the water table, soil, and the vegetation we eat.
This is poison to your body.

Think about the meats you eat. Cows that are eating the
grains exposed to harmful pesticides and toxic chemicals
with absorb them and pass these toxins onto you the
consumer. Many animals are given drugs when they are
sick and hormones to make them grow bigger faster, all
of which end up in the food we eat. They don't just disap-
pear.

We know acid rain kills aquatic life, but how do the levels
affect the consumer when the fish get some toxins, but

not enough to kill them? Do you see what I'm saying here? It's a very gray area that makes us think.

We are destroying our protective ozone layer which is thinning as we speak, allowing dangerous UV rays to seep through that we aren't conditioned to deal with. Sensitive plants and animals are being damaged and destroyed, at what point will we be damaged beyond repair?

Super toxic chemicals are chemicals like dioxins which are simply by-products of industry, and the burning of various toxic chemicals. It's these super chemicals that are the most dangerous to humans, deadly in trace amounts. What happens is they unknowingly enter your body through the food chain, hide out in your fat tissues and cause interference, including genetic mutation and various cancers.

Practical Actions to Take . . .
* Wash all fruits and vegetables thoroughly
* Avoid using harmful chemical cleaning products
* Eat organic fruits and vegetables
* Eat free-range meats that are hormone-free
* Steer clear of processed and packaged foods
* Choose natural and wholesome always
* Don't swim in water near industry or exposed to dangerous chemicals
* Make sure you know the ingredients in your soaps, shampoos, face creams and cosmetics

My Thoughts . . .
With advancement comes more toxins and environmental damage, some experts agree this is the price or progress. Humans are greedy and regardless of the consequences we want more, more, more. If you buy a fancy new car you're adding to the poisonous toxins in

16

our environment, minutely or otherwise. Running your old clunker into the ground is also causing more harmful chemicals to infiltrate into our ecosystem, which eventually is transferred to each one of us in some shape or form, through the foods we eat, the air we breathe, and even the face cream we use.

This is something we are all consciously aware of, yet we really don't seem to care too much about it. Maybe the thought of the consequences of all these serious environmental pollutants is too much to swallow. Particularly since we as humans are the problem. The earth doesn't natural create massive amounts of toxic fumes and poison the atmosphere and all living things. We do.
It's time to do what we can to take action and taking steps towards Clean Eating is definitely a move in the right direction. Agreed?

Toxins and Your Health

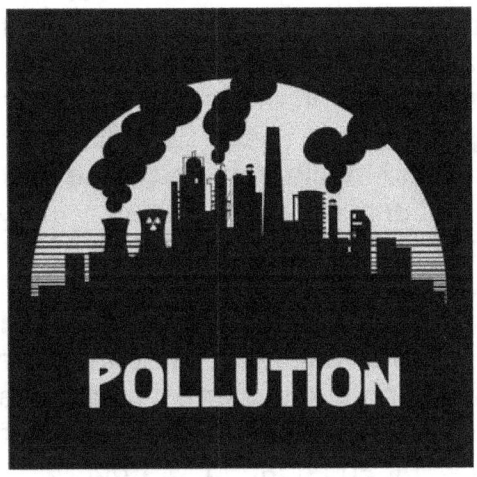

We recognize that we absorb, eat, drink and breathe toxins knowingly or not every day. They surround us and
over time affect each one of us negatively. It's more often
than not, eventually manifesting into disease, and illness
that eventually takes us down, or in the least causes us
huge stress and pain.

Understanding "how" these unnatural chemicals cause
issue with our health is going to give us the desire to take
action and look towards prevention. If we can learn to
avoid toxins in general, this is only going to help up lead
"cleaner" lives with less health issues and a whole lot
more smiles.

Every day we inhale the dangers of cigarette smoke,
truck fumes and industrial waste, spewed carelessly into
the air we breathe in hopes that it will just go away. The

water we drink has been overdosed with chemicals to make it "safe." These poisons make their way into the foods we eat through toxic soils.

Our body is naturally programmed to get rid of "reasonable" waste, but not to the levels and composition we propose today. Your kidneys, liver and lymphatic system works tirelessly to get rid of these extremely dangerous substances, but just can't keep up. This in itself, is jeopardizing your good health because these excess stresses are causing malfunction and inefficiency in your bodily "waste disposal" systems.

The result is these toxins start to build up and poison your organs and internal systems from the inside out, weakening your immune system, causing interference with your intricately functioning internal systems, making you sick and weak and headed for trouble.

If your body is broken down and weak, defenseless, what do you think happens? In simplistic terms you get sick and stay sick because your body has lost the ability to fight disease and make you better.

Your health matters and if you want to take action you are going to have to make a Clean Eating Blueprint. It's your choice.

More Suggestive Tips to Avoid Environmental Toxins
* Eat more fiber so you can naturally remove toxins from your system and function more efficiently
* Drink lots of filtered, bottled or distilled water
* Implement regular detox and "clean" eating strategies
* Ensure effective ventilation and air circulation in your home and workplace
* Wear a mask and other protective wear when painting or cleaning with unnatural substances

* Use all-natural non-toxin cleaners
* Ensure your cosmetics and other personal care creams are safe and all-natural
* Eat organic and clean
* Avoid processed and packaged foods
* Make sure your medications and prescriptions are as "all-natural" as possible

How Do Environmental toxins affect your body?
Each environmental toxin will cause varying issues for each person. What may make one individual deathly ill, might just cause tummy upset in another. Let's have a look at all toxins in general and how they affect the body so we can better understand the big picture, which is taking action to move you towards clean living.

Mercury
Mercury is a metal that naturally occurs in nature, found in water, the soil and air. Microorganisms also transport it into the food chain for consumption. This gets transferred to items we eat like fish, which then causes issue to our health because we eat these fish. I'm sure you've heard on the news or read in the papers about dangerous levels of mercury in specific kinds of fish.

This poison in excess amounts can damage your kidneys and directly affect the nervous system causing issues with coordination, thinking, hearing, vision and may also cause irreversible brain damage.

Action Step - Avoiding fish and other food items with high levels of mercury is something you can do to steer clear of mercury specifically, with all environmental toxins awareness if the first factor. If you are aware, you can minimize exposure and avoid.

Animal Venom

Venom is another natural toxin that may cause a mild or deadly result. You may get a sting from a jelly fish and just get a bit of a burn on your leg or arm. Whereas if you get a bite from a deadly snake and don't seek treatment immediately, you could die.

Action Step - Of course avoidance here is the key and awareness. If you are allergic to bee stings make sure you've got your "adrenaline" with you just in case. Taking anti-venom if bitten is also effective.

Microorganisms
Microorganisms carry different types of bacteria that are the cause of various infectious diseases. An example is Tuberculosis which targets damage to the lungs, brain, spinal cord and kidneys.

Action Step - Making sure you are up to date with your shots is one route to avoid this sometimes deadly condition caused by this natural toxin.

Common Viruses
Contrary to many beliefs viruses aren't living, but they cause infectious disease regardless. These toxic enzymes attack and destroy healthy cells and multiply. The common flu and AIDS are prime examples.

Action Step - Hand washing and sanitation are great places to start. Making sure you are living a healthy and clean lifestyle and steering clear of others that have a runny nose, cough and other flu-like symptoms. Of course AIDS is not transmittable through touch, but it can be contracted through the exchange of bodily fluids. So safe sex and awareness are of ultimate importance.

My Thoughts . . .

Toxins in general will affect you both mentally and physically, causing issues with sight, hearing, tasting, thinking, motor skills, physical appearance, along with sometimes directly affecting the function of your internal systems, like breathing and swallowing. Depending on what toxins you've been exposed to, in what amount and under what conditions, will determine the consequences, which could be something as mild as an annoying skin rash, to as deadly as respiratory failure, with hundreds of debilitating diseases thrown in between. Most serious disease is inter-linked to deadly toxins we are exposed to through the environment, knowingly or now.

Your best move is to take action and look to first prevent or limit your exposure to toxins and to adopt clean eating and living to do your mind and body right.

Disease and Toxins

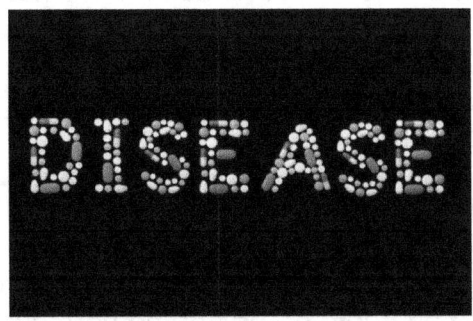

What do you do if you have a headache or other annoying system such as an itchy skin rash? Chances are you probably scoot down to the local pharmacy for some headache tablets or skin cream to make it go away.

What if I told you your headache was being triggered because of specific avoidable toxins you exposed yourself to? What if your annoying skin rash was because of a chemical you were ingesting? This would mean your solution to these ailments is what I term a "band aid" solution. You are just covering up the underlying problem with drugs and other topical measures until and when it surfaces again. It's a method of masking the symptoms or ignoring them, whichever way you choose to look at it.

Over time, this method of dealing with health issues takes its toll. Adding more harmful toxins into your system that you think are helping deal with your current health issues. They are masking the problem and adding more that won't come to surface until years down the road. Accumulated and built up in your internal systems until they start causing serious issues.

It's all about opening your mind here to the best plan of action to control and treat diseases and illnesses you may be battling now and preventing others from entering the picture. Clean eating is one route to better your health and change your direction to improving your health and wellness in the big picture.

Symptoms that you are often experiencing is just your body try to flag down your attention. It wants you to understand these symptoms are just a tiny factor in a much larger issue. You could be poisoning your systems each day by breathing in toxic fumes at work and your body knows if you don't pay attention to the signal, dizziness and headaches each day, these toxins are going to do more than just give you a headache, the damage to your brain will be permanent. This is absolute and there is no turning back when this happens.

By digging further into the root of symptoms of disease you may be experiencing, you are looking to prevent big health issues from developing. Does that make sense?

Toxins are substances that cause mental, emotional, physical and cognitive issues in people.

That said there are two main kinds of toxins we are exposed to regularly:

ENDOGENOUS TOXINS - Toxins that are created because of metabolic imbalances.
EXOGENOUS TOXINS - Toxins that arise from our environment.

Examples of *exogenous toxins* are:

26

* Household water, formaldehyde and fuel
* Mercury, lead and aluminum
* Chloroform, smog and pesticides
* Industrial waste, food poisoning
* Preservatives, tobacco, alcohol and coffee
* The flu, herpes and AIDS

If your body receives too much of any symptom it will get stressed and these toxins will interfere with your natural bodily function, causing disease and serious illness, sometimes even death.

One problem is it is really tough to measure the levels of these toxins in your body and at what level they start seriously affecting you.

We do receive ample warning via the body when toxins are building and there are two main methods of delivery. VARIABLE ILLNESS OR NON-SPECIFIC - This is where you have a whole mess of symptoms, but don't really know the actual facts. You may feel tired, sick to your stomach, and have a headache, but don't really know why.

Often these symptoms are brushed off and explained because of lack of sleep or routine daily stress, when in fact this may be your body signaling you that toxins are building in your system and one day they will explode. KNOWN OR SPECIFIC ILLNESS - This is just where you are experiencing specific symptoms and immediately you pin a cause to them. Symptoms like arthritis or migraines. At least we "think" we know the cause.

In past years our bodies have been stressed increasingly trying to process the increase of toxins we introduce into our bodies. The foods we drink, the air we breathe, and products we put on our skin are getting more "chemical" and this is more dangerous for our health. As a society we eat more chemically loaded processed foods, drink more caffeine and move further away from the natural living of our ancestors. What this does is trigger more health issues, symptoms and disease because your body can only protect you and filter so much. It does have a threshold that as a society we have surpassed ten times over.

Chemicals and toxins are everywhere you look. They are around you, in you, on you and beside you. Talk about overwhelming your protective bodily mechanisms. Just picture someone afraid of water, sitting on a rock in the middle of the ocean as the tide is coming in. It's information overload. There's no place to go, no place to hide, hands are tied, and there is no clear cut positive action that can be taken.

Well when it comes to toxins and your health, your body feels the exact same way as that poor little guy does. Don't you think it's time for us to pull the plug and at least try and drain some of that water away so it's not so depressing and absolute? With clean eating and looking to make cleaner life choices, you are going to give your body a chance to make progress, to help move your health out of the dark and into the light. To reduce the health symptoms, you are suffering because of extreme toxins in general and move your energy levels up, weight down, immune system function into a stronger zone, and help your internal systems as a whole function optimally.

By removing or at least reducing your unified exposure to toxins, you're going to decrease annoying health issues and prevent serious ones from manifesting and stealing your life from you. Having a Clean Eating Blueprint is your first step.

My Thoughts
Each person is different and your body will react to toxins the same. The degree to which you are exposed, how often, the efficiency of your internal filters, and how much you can tolerate the specific substance are factors in determining if the specific toxin is going to mildly affect you or kill you in time.

It may be impossible to know every single toxin entering your system on a daily basis, but you can take action. By first taking the time to become aware of these toxins, and secondly taking measures to reduce or remove them from your system for good, are smart moves.

Clean your system completely of damage already done, or at least as much as you can is also beneficial. Then of course, arming your body with essential vitamins and minerals through Clean Eating that are going to help protect you and give you the healthy energy you need to thrive. The Clean Eating Blueprint does this for you. It gives you a solid base and life perspective that is only going to better your health from what it is today. Looking to better you means you are. You are important and that's non-negotiable. Time for you to get "clean" don't you think?

Action Plan

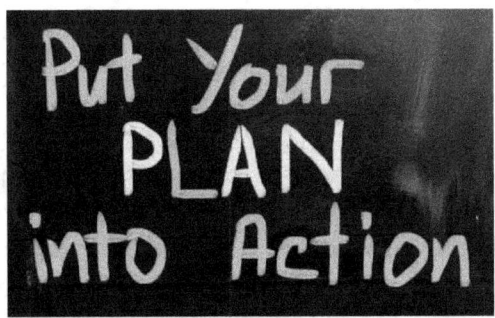

You now have the basis behind what sort of toxins your body has been exposed to and the effects of this on your health and wellness. By removing these poisons building in your internal systems and arming your body with powerful and nutritious nutrients, you are going to be able to restore your health, prevent serious disease and lose weight. Out with the bad and in with the good sounds like a great plan of action, which fits in perfectly with the Clean Eating Blueprint, where you are going to detoxify, restore and re-energize your mind and body so you can get back to clean and healthy living for the long-term.

Clean eating involves two liquid meals a day and one solid, preferably the liquid for breakfast and dinner because this encourages fat breakdown, although it's not the end of the world if you have to mix them up on occasion. Often a smoothie is recommended for breakfast and a smoothie or healthy soup for dinner. It's critical to leave 12 hours between dinner and breakfast because this gives your body the chance to breathe and detoxify while you sleep. Healthy eating is important because otherwise

you are just filling your body full of more toxins and interfering with your good health. It's definitely a no-win
scenario.

Foods Not Allowed
 Processed and fried foods, sugar, caffeine, alcohol,
dairy, red meat, soy, flour and gluten

Make sure you support yourself by getting all the vitamins
and nutrients your body needs, minus toxins and excess
fat. Soups are great because they usually have less calories and fats and protein. Snacks are okay to make sure
you get all the nutrients you need throughout the day.

When it comes to the amount you eat, it's important you
listen to your body and adjust as needed. If you exercise
more, you might need another bowl of soup at dinner and
a few extra vitamin rich snacks throughout the day. It's
important you learn to adjust your eating so that you are
just full and not over-stuffed.

It's important to enjoy your eating. To do this you can always add whatever veggies you need to for a tasty salad.
Slipping in a little extra protein or healthy grains to your
meals is also going to make you smile.

Sample Eating
For the liquid meals you have the ability to use a pre-
made powder formula or create meals. The liquid meals
need to have plenty of fiber and protein, with some good
carbs for energy long-term. The same idea goes with
your solid meal of the day. You want it low-fat with lots of
fresh fruits and veggies, low-fat protein and a healthy
dose of complex carbohydrates. This keeps you eating
healthy and nutritionally, supporting your internal systems
and encouraging easy absorption which is just what your

digestive system craves. This healthy eating also boosts metabolism and this helps your body to burn fat first.

Did You Know? You have to eat to lose weight and if you don't give your body at least 2-3 servings of protein per day, if your body isn't getting enough of this essential macronutrient, it will actually start breaking down your fat burning lean muscle for energy, which of course isn't going to help you one bit because muscle burns more calories than fat, is smaller and more aesthetically pleasing, takes up less space, is firmer than "jiggly" fat, and most importantly you need muscle to stay strong and zap fat.

* Drinking plenty of clean water, green tea and other herbal teas are important for keeping your system hydrated and flushing toxins from your body.

Breakfast/Dinner Smoothies
Energy Booster
6 oz distilled water
1/2 cup low-fat almond milk
1/2 cup avocado
1 scoop all-natural protein powder
1 tbsp flaxseed
1 apple
Approximately 400 calories

Packs a Punch
2 cups spinach
1 carrot
1 cup berries
1 tbsp coconut oil
1 tbsp flaxseed
1 zucchini
3/4 cup almond milk
1 date or drizzle of natural honey to sweeten

1 tbsp wheat germ
Approximately 550 calories

Sweet Sensation
1 nectarine
1 orange
1 mango (peeled)
1 cup almond or rice milk
1/2 cup ice
1 scoop protein powder
1 tbsp flaxseed
Approximately 500 calories

Green N' Delicious
2 cups spinach
1 cup Romaine
1 cucumber
2 celery stalks
1 cup cantaloupe
1 cup honeydew melon
1/2 cup green tea
1 scoop protein powder
1 tbsp flax seed
1 tsp lemon juice
Approximately 500 calories

Nutty Delight
1 cup nuts (almonds, walnuts, pecans)
1/2 cup rice or almond milk
2 cups berries
1/2 peach
1/2 pear
1 scoop protein powder
Approximately 600 calories

Chicken Vegetable Soup
2 cups all natural chicken stock

1 grilled chicken breast chopped
1/2 onion sliced
1 clove garlic minced
1 carrot chopped
1 celery stalk chopped
1 cup broccoli
1 sweet potato chopped
1 cup fresh peas
1/2 cup corn
3/4 cup kidney beans
1 red pepper finely chopped
1/2 cup quinoa

Directions - Simmer all ingredients on med-low for 30 minutes, salt and pepper to taste
Approximately 600 calories

Lunches
Grilled Chicken, Steamed Veggies and Quinoa
Grill chicken and brush with coconut oil, herbs, salt and pepper
Grill onions, zucchini, peppers, carrots, 1 sweet potato (thickly sliced), broccoli
1 cup quinoa prepared as instructed
1 cup fresh berries sprinkled with 1/4 crushed almonds
Green Tea
Water
Approximately 650 calories

Baked Salmon Steak, Spinach Citrus Salad, Whole Grain Rice
1 portion wild salmon baked, brush with olive oil, herbs and spices as desired
3/4 cup whole grain rice
2 cups spinach, tomatoes, cucumber, celery, 1/2 orange, 1/2 grapefruit, 1/2 apple thinly sliced, drizzle good fat dressing

Approximately 600 calories

Vegetarian Orange Salad with a Twist, Steamed Veggies, Whole Grain Bread
2 cups Romaine, 1 orange peeled and sliced, 1/4 cup raisins, 1/4 cup dried cranberries, 1 tsp sunflower seeds, 1 tsp pumpkin seeds, 1/2 cucumber sliced, 1/2 red pepper sliced, 1 tsp flax seed, drizzle good fat salad dressing
1 cup quinoa
Steamed cauliflower, eggplant, spinach, broccoli, buck Choy, parsnip, 1/4 cup slivered almonds
Green Tea
Water
Approximately 600 calories

Note: Nobody wants to be measuring foods and calculating portions. With CLEAN eating what's important is finding what works for you. When a salad includes carrots for instance, add what you like. 1/4 cup shredded would make sense. Most often when a food is mentioned you would use a standard serving. When it comes to fruits and veggies, if you want more and you're hungry just add more! In other words listen to your body and use common sense. Eating should be a science, but rather an experience. A little calculated when you are trying to lose weight, but YOU STILL HAVE CONTROL!

If a lunch menu calls for an apple and you LOVE apples, then have two! Here is a guide for portion control if you are unfamiliar. Use this to find out what amount work for you.

**Meats - 1 portion = size of a deck of cards
Fruit - 1 portion = one piece or 1/2 - 3/4 cup
Vegetables - 1 portion = usually about a cup
Whole Grain Rice/Pasta - I portion = 3/4 cup**

Whole Grain Bread - I portion = 1 slice, Bagel = 1/2 bagel
Whole Grain Cereal - 1 portion = 3/4 - 1 cup
Salad Dressing - 1 portion = 1-2 tbsp (drizzle is best)
Almond/Rice Milk - 1 portion = 1 cup

I think you get the idea. When you are eating healthy, if you are hungry and want a little more, have it. If you are full, eat less. Losing weight and getting healthy is a give and take relationship, and the sooner you start listening to your body and using your noggin, the sooner you are going to reach your goals with a smile. What works for you, works for you and not Mary, Timmy, Johnny or Jenna!

THE THREE MAIN FACTORS IN CLEAN EATING EVERY DAY ARE:

Detoxify
Here you want to get rid of the toxins in your body. By avoiding unhealthy processed and packaged foods, choosing to eat natural and wholesome organic foods and getting rid of bad bacterial in your intestinal system you will remove the barrier for overall good health.

Restore
Now it's time for you to fill your system back up with CLEAN foods that are going to give you all the critical macro and micronutrients your body needs to function optimally. Focusing on supplying your systems with a balance of lean meats, healthy carbs, good fats and all the essential vitamins and minerals your systems depend on, you WILL lose fat and build your body healthy and strong. Better able to resist disease and function at a higher level consistently.

Lots of fresh vegetables and fruits and adequate amounts of lean meats, seeds, nuts and other healthy nutrients are choices you need to make. Foods you need to slowly incorporate into your diet to make your new "normal."

Re-energize

Here is where you get to take positive action above the routine measures to help your body run smoothly and cleanly. Some may think of these actions as luxurious, but I would rather view them as "better" and "preventative."

By taking time to better your mind through meditation and scheduling regular saunas for instance to help enhance the detox process, you WILL be on target to zap excess fat, unleash hidden energy and strengthen both your mind and body positively to better absorb daily life challenges. The mind is a powerful thing and if you "think" it you can do it.

My Thoughts . . .
Taking action is what it's all about. Using the best information you have that will help you to detoxify, restore and re-energize your body so that all your systems can run "clean." It's all about getting rid of the toxins that are slowing your down and in actuality slowly poisoning you, then giving back to your body the "right" vitamins and minerals it needs to service you. Making better and healthier food choices is going to do this.

Finally you get to take your health to the next level by energizing your mind and body. Making sure you are always moving towards that healthy life balance we all crave; mind, body and soul. The one where you are feel-

ing strong and your body is void of disease. Your heart and lungs are working effectively and efficiently pumping clean nutrients throughout your internal systems because you are making natural and wholesome eating choices, eliminating deadly processed and packaged foods and exercising enough to at least break a sweat.
Bigger and better is just around the corner and by taking action with the Clean Eating Blueprint you are creating a map, through some trial and error, to awesome health!

40

Clean Eating Benefits

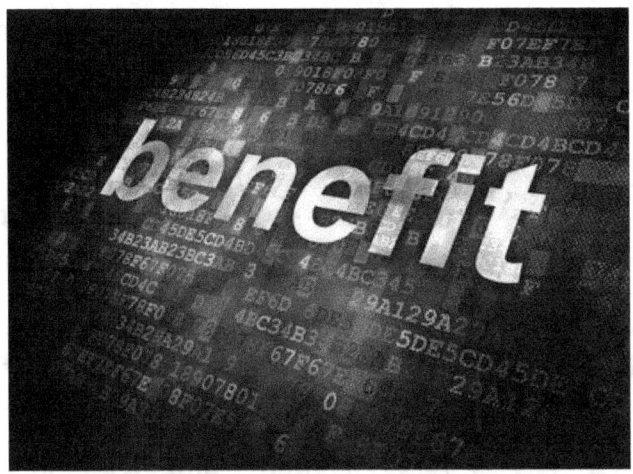

Clean eating is often discredited by people because they are afraid of moving away from what they know and are conditioned to eat, accept there is a better way, and take action to "re-learn" how to eat.

There is no question that the eating practiced of people 500 years ago was much healthier than today. The difference is in the convenience. For the price of convenience today, we pay the price of good health.

Think about it . . .
Processed and packaged high-fat, low nutrient foods are a staple for us. Why? Well because we always want it faster, faster, faster! This is a dangerous theory of eating because the sugar refined foods we are eating are extremely addictive. More so, if we choose to have a sweet

on an empty stomach because this tells our body that whenever we are hungry we should crave sugar.

Who's to blame? Who Cares?
You can blame progress, extreme life stress, our parents, fast-food restaurants, greedy money hungry people . . .

It really doesn't matter. You get to choose to open your mind to change or close the door shut, not even try and look forward to a fat and unhealthy life that's going to full of depression, pain, frustration and an early death.

You can try. You can use the Clean Eating Blueprint strategy as a base for building a leaner, stronger, healthier and happier you. It's YOUR choice!

By choosing to remove built up harmful toxins and eat energizing, nutrient dense, metabolic boosting foods always, you are only going to get "better." Here are some of the advantages that come with the "better" choice . . .

Weight Loss or Gain
Lower Blood Pressure
Lower Cholesterol
Increased Energy
Clearer Thinking
Improved Self-Confidence
Eating Satisfaction
Stronger Immune System
Healthier Digestive Process
Weight Stabilization Long-Term
Stable Blood Sugars
Decreased Mood Swings
Improved Physical Appearance
Healthier Hair, Nails and Skin
Longer Living

Increased Mobility and Motility
Less Risk for Serious Disease
Increased Optimism
Less stress

My Thoughts . . .
I don't know about you, but this list looks pretty inviting to me. The issue with most people isn't that they don't WANT to make health changes for the better. Sometimes it's not even the fact they don't know how. It's the effort to get started, to admit there's a better way and to actually get themselves on a routine of CHANGE that's the toughest. Habits are hard to break.

First thing you have to do if you are going to be success-ful in better health with the help of Clean Eating Blueprint is you MUST commit to doing everything possible to set yourself up for success. This is going to take . . .

* Effort
* Give and take
* Open Mind
* Perseverance
* WILLINGNESS to change
* Acceptance of screwing up
* Letting go of past mistakes
* Getting back up and on that crazy horse
A COMMITMENT TO YOUR GOOD HEALTH THAT YOU WILL NEVER QUIT ON.

The choice is yours - do it or don't, but whatever you do don't nitpick and complain about it . . . Just Do It!

Benefits of Exercise

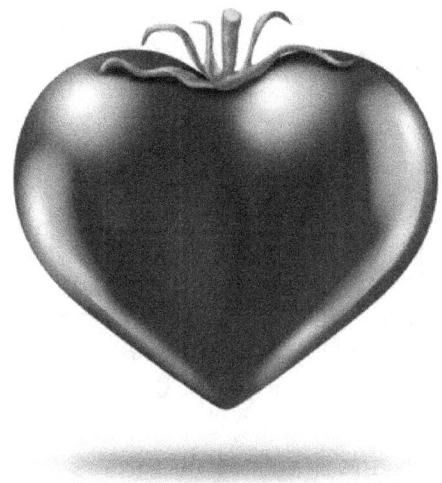

Something you need to accept if you haven't already is that regular DAILY physical activity is a fact of life. It's something your body was designed and made for. It's you and I through life that have screwed this concept up and opted for disgustingly obvious laziness.

Could you imagine what would have happened to man 500 years ago if a lion decided it wanted to eat him for lunch and this poor man had trouble getting off the couch because he was 50 pounds overweight and halfway through his family sized bag of chips and -extra- large chocolate shake?

My totally overdone point here is that man wasn't born with "progress" and convenience at his fingertips. Physical energy was required for mere survival. If you couldn't run you definitely wouldn't be eating. If you weren't in fantastic cardiovascular shape and didn't have muscles like a truck you most certainly would eventually become lunch for some sort of dangerous predator. If not you would get sick and die because there was no medicine available to bandage diseases and illnesses. Do you get what I'm saying here?

Time for us to re-program our minds and body's to fit regular physical exercise into our day, which will help speed up the weight loss results we will get through clean eating. It's a group effort here and even if you just start by fitting an hour walk in each day you are one step closer to "better." Committing to pushing yourself to improve your lung capacity and muscle strength continuously is only going to get you the results you are looking for faster. Isn't that what you want?
Leaner, slimmer, stronger, healthier - faster?

Here's what you need -
45 min - 1 hour cardiovascular exercise daily
15-20 min strength training or weight lifting 2-3 times a week

The Benefits of Cardiovascular Exercise
* Lose weight
* Maintain weight
* Decrease risk of serious disease
* Improve cognitive function
* Improve circulation
* Regulate bowel movements
* Remove toxins
* Release "feel good" endorphins
* Trigger optimism
* Lower stress
* Increase metabolism

* Lower blood pressure and cholesterol
Examples
* Fast walking
* Biking or hiking
* Swimming
* Boot camp classes
* Aerobic classes
* Skiing
* Running
* Tennis, basketball, squash or any other racket sport
* Roller-skating or rollerblading
* Ice skating or hockey
* Aqua aerobics
* Dance class

The Benefits of Muscle Building
* Increased energy
* More calories burned than fat
* Less effort more energy used
* Improved athletic performance
* Decreases effects of sarcopenia (natural muscle loss)
* Improved self-confidence
* Increased blood flow
* Attracts positive attention (muscle just looks "hot!")
* Less aches and pains
* Decreased risk of bodily injury

Examples
* Weight machines gym
* Weight bands
* Body resistance (pushups, sit-ups, squats)
* Free weights
* Boot camp classes (weights/strength training and cardio combined)

Note 1 - Muscles can be built at any age, whether you're twenty or ninety. Of course, always check with your doctor first before starting an exercise regimen. Note 2 - Interval Training is the fastest and most effective way to lose weight and build your body strong. Alternating between bouts of cardiovascular exercise and weight training will keep your body and mind guessing, maximizing the energy burned. Diversity is key so changing the pace, frequency, rep count, intensity and duration of each exercise activity is going to get your fantastic results fast!

My Thoughts . .
Exercising is something your mind and body needs. Start slow and work your way up to make it enjoyable and ensure you don't injure yourself. If you need to start by just walking for 45 minutes each day, then do it. Gradually increase the pace and then start changing things up. Maybe go for a bike ride for 20 minutes and then walk for the remainder. Add some weights into the mix and you are only getting closer to your goal faster of losing weight and getting healthy for life. It's going to stick because you are setting yourself up for success and doing it the "right" way.

The "Big" Picture

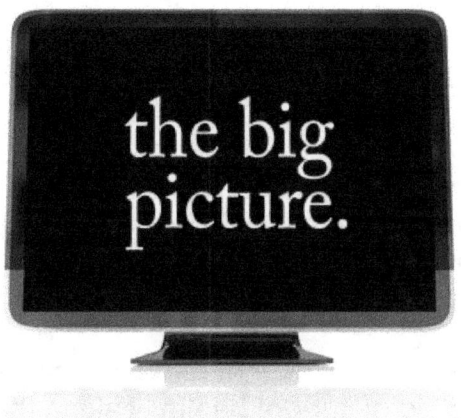

Your good health is the most valuable asset you have. Without it, you have nothing.

This means it only makes sense that you do everything you can within reasons to build your mind and body healthy and strong, to lose fat and keep your body at its optimal weight so that your systems can work better and better. Good health isn't a one stop shop. You don't decide on an eating, exercise, and lifestyle routine and expect it to last forever, just as life is ever-changing so is your body. Diversity is the key to results.

Clean Eating Blueprint is a proven evolutionary science based "lifestyle" strategy that's only going to better you. Helping you zap fat fast, gain energy and confidence, avoid disease, decrease chronic symptoms and flip your switch to positive.

Removing all the negative (toxins, chemicals, preservatives, excess fats) from your systems gives your body and mind a chance to strip down to "normal" and rebuild.

Understanding having to avoid serious toxins in and around you is the first step in preventing sickness and disease.

Taking Action in making sure you minimize your exposure to environmental hazards in the air, food and in skin products is also critical if you want to give your body a chance to run smoothly without interference.

Implementing strategies that make sense to you are important in the big picture of health. Taking the time to make better food choices that are natural and wholesome is important. Slowly getting rid of bad fast-food and processed eating habits and replenishing them with what nature intended. Looking to eat healthy food choices in the "right" portions is also important in setting yourself up for results, losing fat quickly and sensibly through great eating and exercise so that you can live clean for life.

Exercising is most definitely critical in good health and is often downplayed or totally ignored in popular eating strategies. Your body is working hard and always burning energy and to take care of it you need to get regular muscle building and cardiovascular activity simply because this is a part of clean health. Think of it as leaving your bike out in the rain for a year without use. What happens to it? Well it rusts and doesn't work very well when you want to take it for a spin. It's the same thing with your body. Take care of it and keep it strong with a good exercise regimen and it's only going to serve you better.

Find your balance in exercise activities you like, keep it diverse and always challenging and everything you desire in good health is only going to surface sooner. Start slow and always look to improve and before you know it you won't even have to think about exercising because it will just be a part of your normal daily routine, for all the right reasons.

Take care of your mental by de-stressing regularly with meditation, yoga, a sauna, or massage for example.
By giving your body the chance to relax and de-stress, you are restoring your systems to their ultimate power level, opening your internal energy channels and letting your body run more efficiently. That means a happier, leaner and healthier you.

Experts agree that natural is better and this means the way people lived a thousand years ago, before "industrial progress" came into place, were a heck of a lot healthier than we are today.
Why?

Simply because they didn't know any better than to listen to their body and give it what it needed as much as they could. Health issues arose because some things just weren't always available in ancient days. There may have been hunger and it was recognized, but if the head tribe member screwed up and lead everyone away from fresh game, then the whole tribe would suffer without food.

They didn't have the choice we have today when hunger strikes of ten zillion fast food restaurants within reach. It's an exaggeration I know, but a solid point nonetheless.

People in days past never took food for granted. They were overjoyed to eat a fresh antelope or bison with wild berries and field grass, when there was food to eat they would feast until they couldn't eat another bite. The difference is they were always giving the body exactly what it needs nutritionally to run top notch. Overeating was never a bad thing, because they lived in a world where the strongest survived, if you wanted to live you had to build your body and mind strong, making sure you got enough to eat and lots of rest to restore your natural bodily systems. Your life depended on it.

Today there are huge consequences with overeating, obesity, disease and illness to start. By not eating "clean" we are poisoning our bodies by doing what is natural to us, the act of eating. We create huge interference with the bad food choices we have created and this negatively affects us mentally, physically, socially and emotionally.

WE have created this only YOU can decide to change it. If you truly want to live your life lean and strong, if you really want to better your health on all levels and feel energized and alive, strong and happy, then YOU need to learn about, understand and apply the basic principles of Clean Eating Blueprint to your life. Take it one step at a time. Just put one foot in front of the other all eyes forward. Look at the Big Picture of life and apply.

Final Thoughts . . .

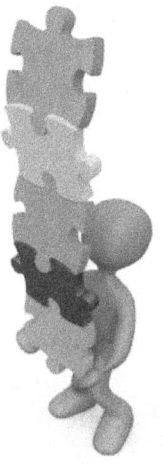

It should be because your health will determine your quality and length of life. If you want to live a long time and experience all the wonders of our world, good and bad, you need to take care of your health. Treat it with respect. Take the time to do maintenance and always look to strengthening and improving it to the best of your abilities.

Understanding what your body needs and what it doesn't need to run well is very important. Clean eating is a very basic principle that everyone was born with. Making sure we live as close as we reasonably can with nature means you are giving your "self" what it requires to last longer and make you happier.

We have poisoned our environment over time and this has not only caused stress on all living organisms, it has also interfered with the healthy fuel we rely on for life. Water and food sources from the earth are tainted with toxins that we eventually ingest. This causes more interference with the intricately run internal system in each of us. Like a game of dominoes, we create more and more problems, illness, disease and annoying symptoms because we are not living cleanly. The price of progress, I guess.

Are we ever going to be able to remove all toxins from the air we breathe, food we eat, and environment as a whole? It's not likely. What we can do is take action to avoid and eliminate as much as possible so we can lessen the consequences and better our health drastically. Isn't something better than nothing?

Time to Take ACTION . . .

KEY PRINCIPLES TO CLEAN EATING
Keep Tabs on Fat, Salt and Sugar
Removing processed and packaged foods is going to help eliminate most of the fats, sugars and excess salt from your daily eating. Most natural "clean" foods are low in fat, contain little or no sugar, and if they do it's natural and easily absorbed, and little or no salt.

Pick Whole, Natural Foods
Of course, natural foods are foods you would get naturally from the earth and presented that way. This means organic and void of harmful chemicals, toxins and hormones during the growing process. There is a difference between strawberries that have been grown organically and those that have come from a supermarket shelf and have been exposed to pesticides and growth hormones. In other words, not all strawberries are created equal.

Be smart and make sure the foods you are putting in your body are clean.

Watch Your Beverages
The best drink for you is pure water. Water that is distilled, bottle or from a pure spring, void of any sort of chemical processes or toxins added. Unsweetened herbal teas are also a great choice or unsweetened almond or rice milk for example.

Drinking soda just adds loads of sugary nutrition-less calories to your diet, along with all sorts of nasty chemicals. Did you know that Coke can actually clean a blocked feeding tube line out? The citric acid in Coke can also make your toilet squeaky clean!

Your body needs water to work properly, and your brain needs it to function. Six to eight glasses a day minimum is best. Keep it clean as this is also going to help you burn fat and clean the built up toxins from your system.

Avoid Refined Foods and Choose Unrefined
White bread, pasta, rice and sugary sweets does nothing for you nutritionally. Choosing clean and healthy unrefined foods like whole grain pasta, bread, rice, millet and quinoa is going to give you plenty of fiber, loads of nutrients, very little fat and this is just what your body ordered. These complex carbs will also provide longer term energy for you to function with a smile longer, burning more fat and calories than you would otherwise.

Food Combinations
Making sure you get lean protein, complex carbohydrates and some good fats at every meal is going to ensure you have the energy you need to burn off excess fat, improve immunity and build your body and mind strong. The protein will help build lean muscle and the carbs will fuel you

long-term. Fats will help to encourage fat burning and make certain you have the energy you need to get lean and run optimally. Greens come in the picture to help increase your fiber intake which helps to transport toxins through the exit doors.

Regular Exercise
Exercise needs to be a part of your every day. It's going to help you lose weight, get the nutrients to the awaiting organs, and make you feel like a million bucks. Through trial and error you can figure out what sort of exercising makes you smile and make it happen. Diversity is the key as we've discussed and the effort you put in here is exactly what you're going to receive in results.

Work hard at it and you will see fast results. Make excuses and whine about it and you will get nothing. It's your choice.

Clean Eating Blueprint is a lifestyle strategy for those that want to make the most of their life. It's for people that are willing to work hard and make the changes necessary to stop damaging their systems and try and make things right, to clean the slate and re-build it "healthier" and "cleaner."

It's all about finding through trial and error what works for you, even if you take from this book just one positive health change, you are bettering you. Isn't that what life is all about?

Look for the good in everything. Taking bits and pieces of information that makes sense to you and applying it, personalizing it with the goal of self-improvement. Better health, smarter choices and a happier more fulfilled you.

The ball's in your court. It's time for you to take the good with the bad and use the Clean Eating Blueprint to tip you in the direction of positive! Good Luck!

We have the choice to look for the positive or the negative in life. You can choose to lift someone up or to stomp on them. Writing is my passion and I work hard at it, with the goal of helping make people better. If you gain a new piece of knowledge, read something that makes you think, or perhaps even smile a few times, then I am happy and content!

Life's just too short not to tune into optimism. If your glass is half full, then I invite you to read my writing, and if you have a minute to spare when you're through, **I would appreciate your review.** This will help me better myself and my writing. I thank you in advance and appreciate you.